THE COMPLETE PCOS COOKBOOK FOR NEWLY DIAGNOSED

A GUIDE WITH NUTRITIOUS RECIPES TO CONTROL INSULIN RESISTANCE AND ELIMINATE PCOS SYMPTOMS

KAREN EDMONDS

1

TABLE OF CONTENT

INTRODUCTION

Starting a wellness journey after being diagnosed with PCOS presents a difficulty as well as a chance for change. We cordially encourage you to embark on a culinary journey with "The Complete PCOS Cookbook for Newly Diagnosed," which is designed to empower and nourish individuals navigating the complex terrain of polycystic ovarian syndrome. See the cookbook as your go-to friend, a confidante in the kitchen who not only knows the ins and outs of PCOS but also infuses each delicious page with the restorative power of food.

Introducing Karen, a colourful soul who, after being diagnosed with PCOS, found herself at a turning point similar to many others. Frustrated by the dearth of easily accessible materials that fused great food with sound nutritional advice, Karen set out to write a cookbook that would demystify PCOS while also igniting a passion for healthful, delectable meals.

As you explore this cookbook, expect a voyage beyond dishes; it's a story of tenacity, exploration, and delectable victories against obstacles related to PCOS. You'll find a sympathetic companion who comprehends the mental and physical aspects of adjusting to a PCOS-friendly lifestyle through Karen's personal tales. This cookbook is a guide to taking back control, enjoying food, and starting a new chapter in your well-being. It's much more than just a list of recipes. So let's set out on this culinary adventure together, where empowerment and sustenance collide and each meal serves as a springboard to a happier, healthier self.

CHAPTER 1:

UNDERSTANDING PCOS (POLYCYSTIC OVARY SYNDROME)

PCOS, also referred to as polycystic ovary syndrome, is a complicated and widespread hormonal condition that affects people who are assigned to the feminine gender at birth. PCOS is a disorder that causes distinct difficulties for those who are diagnosed with it. It is characterised by a variety of symptoms, such as irregular menstrual periods, elevated levels of male hormones (androgens), and the formation of tiny cysts on the ovaries.

When we explore the complexities of PCOS in the context of a cookbook, it becomes clear that food and hormone balance, play a critical role. This section will shed light on the special opportunities and challenges that come up when creating a cookbook for people who have just received a PCOS diagnosis.

PCOS Nutritional Foundations

Balancing Macros and Micros: The cookbook delves into the macro and micronutrients that are critical for regulating PCOS symptoms, fostering hormonal equilibrium, and bolstering general health.

Dietary Influence on Insulin Resistance: It's Critical to Recognise Insulin's Role in PCOS. The cookbook explains how certain food decisions might lessen insulin resistance, which is a typical PCOS symptom.

A Culinary Philosophy Centred on PCOS

Choosing to Eat Whole Foods: The cookbook informs readers about the advantages of making nutrient-dense dietary choices in managing PCOS and promotes a focus on full, unprocessed foods.

Mindful Eating for Hormonal Harmony: The cookbook promotes mindful eating techniques in addition to recipes, acknowledging the link between stress, hormone balance, and food selections.

Recipes Compliant with PCOS Fundamentals

Variety and Balance: Every dish is designed to provide a consistent energy level and satisfaction by balancing the amounts of healthy fats, carbohydrates, and proteins.

Anti-Inflammatory Ingredients: This section of the cookbook examines the anti-inflammatory qualities of specific foods and presents recipes that aim to lessen inflammation, which is an important factor in the management of PCOS.

Techniques for Meal Planning

Structured Meal Plans: Easy-to-follow meal plans designed specifically for people with PCOS make it easier to prepare well-balanced, PCOS-friendly meals.

Flexibility and Adaptability: Taking into account that every person has different needs, the cookbook provides advice on how to modify recipes to suit a range of dietary restrictions and tastes.

Educating and Empowering

Nutritional Knowledge Hub: The cookbook is more than just a collection of recipes; it's also an instructional resource that promotes knowledge about how nutrition affects hormonal health.

Navigating Food Myths: By dispelling widespread myths, the cookbook gives readers access to fact-based knowledge, enabling them to make well-informed dietary decisions.

PCOS Nutrition Basics

To navigate the difficulties of Polycystic Ovary Syndrome (PCOS), a comprehensive approach to diet is required. This section digs into the core concepts of PCOS nutrition, providing insights into dietary choices that might improve hormonal balance and general health.

Macronutrient Balance

Protein Importance: Investigating the importance of protein in PCOS management, particularly its influence on satiety, muscle health, and hormone control.

Choosing Healthy Fats: Recognise the importance of include omega-3 fatty acids and monounsaturated fats in your diet for inflammation reduction and hormonal support.

Complex Carbohydrates: Emphasising whole grains, legumes, and fiber-rich meals to control blood sugar levels and manage insulin resistance.

Hormonal Health Micronutrients

Vitamins and Minerals: Investigating the role of certain vitamins and minerals crucial to PCOS treatment, such as vitamin D, B-complex vitamins, and minerals such as magnesium and zinc.

Antioxidants and Phytochemicals: Emphasising the need of adding colourful fruits and vegetables in your diet to give a variety of antioxidants and phytochemicals for general health.

PCOS Mindful Eating

Understanding Hunger and Fullness: Promoting mindful eating practises to build a healthy relationship with food while also assisting with weight control and hormonal balance.

Meal Timing and Frequency: Discussing the need of eating regularly to maintain stable blood sugar levels and avoid hormonal changes.

Addressing Insulin Resistance

Low-Glycemic Index Foods: Include low-glycemic index foods and fruits (Green vegetables, grapefruits, cherries, pears, raw carrots, kidney beans, chickpeas and lentils) in your diet to control insulin resistance and lower your risk of type 2 diabetes.

Sugar and Processed Food Impact: Discussing the effect of added sugars and processed foods in worsening insulin resistance and providing alternatives.

PCOS and Hydration

Water Intake: Emphasising the significance of sufficient hydration in supporting metabolic functioning, maintaining skin health, and assisting with weight control.

Herbal Teas and Infusions: Investigating herbal teas that may be beneficial for hormonal balance and stress reduction.

PCOS Nutritional Customization

Individualised Approaches: Recognising that the nutritional needs of people with PCOS vary, and offering advice on how to modify dietary recommendations based on personal preferences and health objectives.

Collaboration with Healthcare Professionals: Encourage interaction with healthcare practitioners or nutrition experts for tailored advice and assistance.

Individuals may establish the groundwork for a well-balanced and individualised dietary strategy that matches with their particular health demands and aids to the optimal treatment of PCOS symptoms by understanding these PCOS nutrition principles.

CHAPTER 2: MEAL PLANNING FOR PCOS

Making nutritious and well-balanced meals is an important part of controlling Polycystic Ovary Syndrome (PCOS). This section describes successful meal planning options that are geared to satisfy the unique nutritional demands associated with PCOS, while also maintaining hormonal balance and general well-being.

Recognising Portion Control and Timing

Portion Guidelines: Providing realistic portion control suggestions to help you manage your calorie intake, assist your weight loss, and address insulin sensitivity.

Meal Timing: Investigating the significance of regular meal intervals and consistent meal timing in order to stabilise blood sugar levels and reduce hormonal swings.

Preparing Well-balanced Meals

Protein-Rich Options: Provide a range of protein sources to maintain muscle health and satiety, such as lean meats, fish, eggs, and plant-based proteins.

Including Healthy Fats: Including sources such as avocados, nuts, seeds, and olive oil to supply needed fatty acids and support hormonal activities.

Emphasising Whole Grains: Whole grains such as quinoa, brown rice, and oats are recommended for their fibre content and capacity to manage blood sugar levels.

Meal Planning and Batch Cooking

Techniques for Efficient Planning: Introducing time-saving meal prep ideas to expedite the cooking process and assure weekly access to nutritious meals.

Batch Cooking for Convenience: Investigating the advantages of batch cooking to have a steady supply of PCOS-friendly meals on hand while minimising dependency on processed foods.

Fiber-Rich and Nutrient-Dense Choices

Vegetables and Fruits: Promote a colourful variety of vegetables and fruits high in fibre, antioxidants, and vitamins to promote digestive health and general wellness.

Legumes and Whole Foods: Including legumes, beans, and whole foods in meals to increase nutritional density and encourage sustained energy.

Fluid Consumption and Hydration

Water as a Priority: Stressing the need of drinking water for hydration, metabolic support, and the promotion of clear skin.

Herbal Teas and Infusions: Introducing alternatives to sugary beverages, such as herbal teas, can help with hydration while also potentially delivering health advantages.

Making Modifications to Traditional Recipes

PCOS-Friendly Swaps: Providing substitutes for popular items in conventional recipes in order to match with PCOS nutritional guidelines while maintaining flavour.

Making Flavorful, Balanced Dishes: Showing how to infuse PCOS-friendly dishes with a range of herbs and spices to improve flavour and enjoyment.

Mindful Eating and Flexibility

Balanced Indulgences: Encourage a balanced attitude to occasional pleasures while maintaining a nutrient-rich and balanced diet overall.

Mindful Eating Practises: Advocate for mindful eating strategies to improve self-awareness during meals and develop a healthy connection with food.

Individuals with PCOS may build a sustainable and pleasurable approach to nutrition by incorporating these meal planning ideas into their everyday lives, supporting their health objectives and improving overall well-being.

CHAPTER 3: PCOS-FRIENDLY RECIPES

Berry Protein Smoothie Bowl

Ingredients:

- 1 cup of mixed berries including strawberries, blueberries, raspberries
- 1/2 cup of Greek yogurt
- 1 scoop of protein powder
- 1/4 cup of granola
- 1 tablespoon of chia seeds
- Nuts (almonds, walnuts) for garnish

Preparation:

- Greek yoghurt, protein powder, and mixed berries should all be blended until smooth.
- Transfer the smoothie into a bowl.
- Top with granola, chia seeds, and a sprinkle of nuts.

Nutritional Value (Approx.):

Calories: 350-400

Protein: 20g

Carbohydrates: 40g

Fat: 15g

Fiber: 8g

Quinoa Breakfast Bowl

Ingredients:

- 1/2 cup of cooked quinoa
- Mixed fresh fruit (berries, banana slices)
- Greek yogurt
- Honey for drizzling

Preparation:

- Follow the directions on the package to cook the quinoa.
- Arrange cooked quinoa, Greek yoghurt, and fresh fruit in a bowl.
- Pour some honey over it.

Nutritional Value (Approx.):

Calories: 300-350

Protein: 10g

Carbohydrates: 50g

Fat: 5g

Fiber: 7g

Whole Grain Pancakes and Waffles

Whole Grain Pancakes:

Ingredients:

- 1 cup of whole wheat flour
- 1 tablespoon of sugar
- 1 teaspoon of baking powder
- 1/2 teaspoon of baking soda
- 1/4 teaspoon salt
- 1 cup of buttermilk
- 1 large egg
- 2 tablespoons of melted butter or oil
- 1 teaspoon vanilla extract

Preparation:

- In a big bowl, mix together the whole wheat flour, sugar, baking powder, baking soda, and salt.
- In a separate bowl, whisk together the buttermilk, egg, melted butter or oil, and vanilla extract.
- Pour the wet ingredients into the dry ingredients and stir until just combined. Do not overmix; lumps are okay.
- Grease a non-stick skillet or griddle with cooking spray or butter and heat it over medium heat.
- For each pancake, pour 1/4 cup of batter onto the griddle.
- Cook until bubbles form on the surface, then flip and cook until the other side is golden brown.
- Serve with your favorite toppings such as fresh berries, maple syrup, or a dollop of Greek yogurt.

Nutritional Value (Approx. per serving):

Calories: 150-180

Protein: 5g

Carbohydrates: 25g

Fat: 5g

Fiber: 3g

Whole Grain Waffles:

Ingredients:

- 1 cup of whole wheat flour
- 1 tablespoon of sugar
- 1 teaspoon of baking powder
- 1/2 teaspoon of baking soda
- 1/4 teaspoon of salt
- 1 cup of buttermilk
- 1 large egg
- 2 tablespoons of melted butter or oil
- 1 teaspoon vanilla extract

Preparation:

- As directed by the manufacturer, preheat your waffle iron.
- In a big bowl, mix together the whole wheat flour, sugar, baking powder, baking soda, and salt.

- In a separate bowl, whisk together the buttermilk, egg, melted butter or oil, and vanilla extract.
- Pour the wet ingredients into the dry ingredients and stir until just combined.
- Lightly grease the waffle iron with cooking spray or butter.
- Once the waffle iron grid is covered, pour enough batter over it and cover it.
- Cook in accordance with the waffle iron's instructions until crisp and golden brown.
- Serve the waffles with your favorite toppings, such as fresh fruit, yogurt, or a drizzle of honey.

Nutritional Value (Approx. per serving):

Calories: 180-220

Protein: 6g

Carbohydrates: 30g

Fat: 7g

Fiber: 4g

CHAPTER 4: LUNCH AND DINNER OPTIONS

Mango Avocado Quinoa Salad

Ingredients:

- 1 cup of cooked quinoa
- 1 ripe mango, diced
- 1 avocado, diced
- Cherry tomatoes, halved
- Red onion, finely cut
- Fresh cilantro, chopped
- Lime vinaigrette dressing (lime juice, olive oil, honey, salt, and pepper)

Preparation:

- In a sizable bowl, combine quinoa, mango, avocado, cherry tomatoes, red onion, and cilantro.
- Drizzle with lime vinaigrette dressing and toss gently.

Nutritional Value (Approx.):

Calories: 400-450

Protein: 7g

Carbohydrates: 55g

Fat: 20g

Fiber: 10g

Turkey and Quinoa Stuffed Bell Peppers

Ingredients:

- Bell peppers cut in half, with seeds removed
- Lean ground turkey
- Cooked quinoa
- Black beans, drained and rinsed
- Diced tomatoes
- Onion, diced
- Mexican spices (cumin, chili powder, paprika)
- Shredded cheese (optional)

Preparation:

- Set oven temperature to 375°F, or 190°C.
- Cook the ground turkey, onion, and spices in a pan until browned.
- Add the diced tomatoes, cooked quinoa, and black beans.
- Place the mixture of turkey and quinoa inside bell peppers.
- Add some shredded cheese on top, if desired.
- Bake until peppers are soft.

Nutritional Value (Approx.):

Calories: 350-400

Protein: 25g

Carbohydrates: 30g

Fat: 15g

Fiber: 8g

Vegetarian Lentil Curry

Ingredients:

- Lentils, cooked
- 13.5 oz canned Coconut milk
- 1 Onion, diced
- 3 cloves of Garlic, minced
- Ginger, grated
- 1 ½ tablespoon of Curry powder
- ½ tablespoon of Turmeric
- Spinach leaves
- 1 ½ Tomatoes, diced
- One handful of Cilantro, chopped
- Brown rice for serving

Preparation:

- Sauté the ginger, garlic, and onion in a pot until they become tender.
- Stir in the turmeric and curry powder.
- Add the cooked lentils, tomatoes, and spinach after adding the coconut milk.
- Simmer for the flavours to combine.
- Serve with cilantro on top of brown rice.

Nutritional Value (Approx.):

Calories: 350-400

Protein: 15g

Carbohydrates: 50g

Fat: 10g

Fiber: 12g

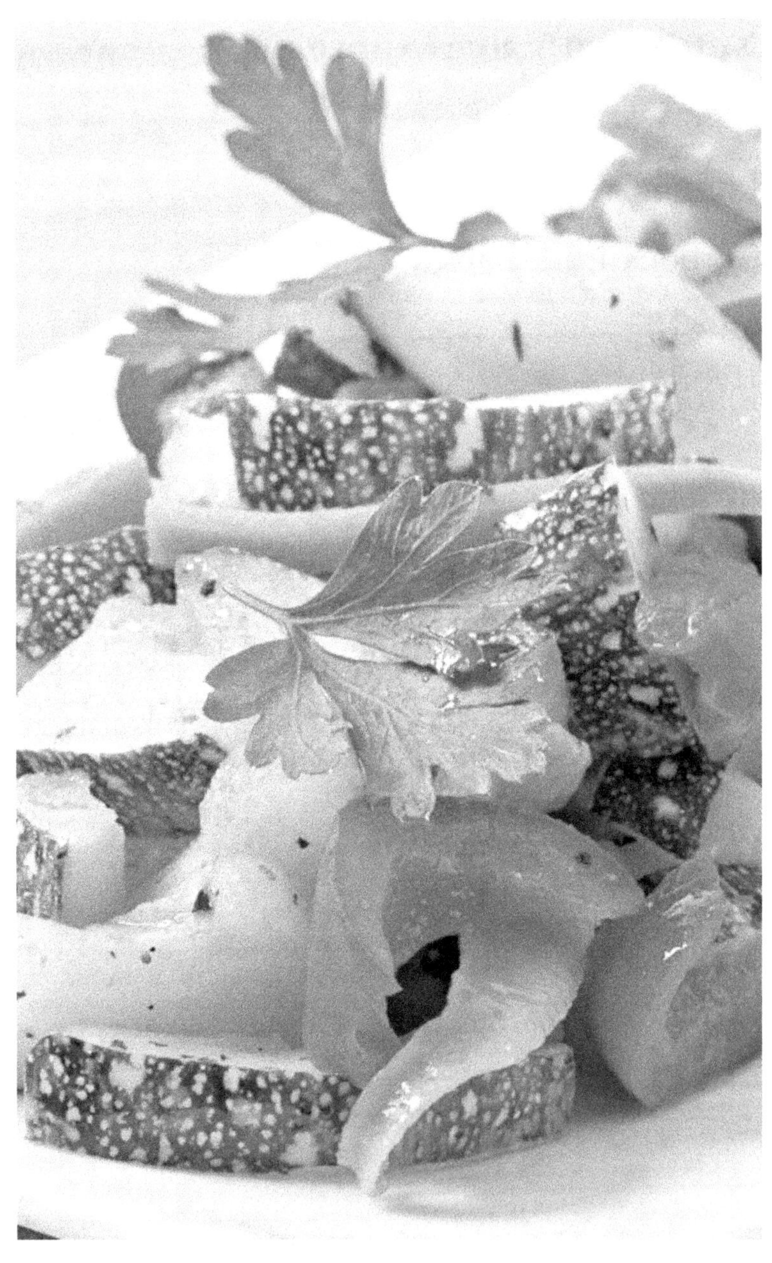

CHAPTER 5: SNACKS AND DESSERTS

Cottage Cheese and Pineapple Bowl

Ingredients:

- 1 cup low-fat cottage cheese
- Fresh pineapple chunks
- Mint leaves for garnish

Preparation:

- Mix cottage cheese and fresh pineapple chunks in a bowl.
- Garnish with mint leaves.

Nutritional Value (Approx. per serving):

Calories: 200-250

Protein: 20g

Carbohydrates: 25g

Fat: 5g

Fiber: 2g

Vegetable Sticks with Hummus

Ingredients:

- Carrot sticks
- Cucumber slices
- Bell pepper strips
- Hummus for dipping

Preparation:

- Wash and cut vegetables into sticks or slices.
- Serve with hummus for a satisfying and nutrient-packed snack.

Nutritional Value (Approx. per serving):

Calories: 150-200

Protein: 5g

Carbohydrates: 20g

Fat: 8g

Fiber: 5g

Almond Butter Banana Bites

Ingredients:

- Bananas, sliced
- Almond butter
- Chia seeds or shredded coconut for coating

Preparation:

- Drizzle banana slices with almond butter.
- To give more texture, roll in shredded coconut or chia seeds.
- Chill in the fridge prior to serving.

Nutritional Value (Approx. per serving):

Calories: 150-180

Protein: 4g

Carbohydrates: 20g

Fat: 8g

Fiber: 3g

Pumpkin Oatmeal Cookies:

Ingredients:

- 1 cup canned pumpkin
- 2 cups of rolled oats
- 1/2 cup of maple syrup
- 1/4 cup of coconut oil
- 1 teaspoon of vanilla extract
- Pumpkin pie spice (cinnamon, nutmeg, cloves)

Preparation:

- Combine canned pumpkin, rolled oats, maple syrup, melted coconut oil, vanilla extract, and pumpkin pie spice in a bowl.
- Using a fork, flatten the spoonfuls that are placed onto a baking sheet.
- Bake for 12 to 15 minutes at 350°F (175°C).

Nutritional Value (Approx. per serving):

Calories: 120-150

Protein: 2g

Carbohydrates: 20g

Fat: 5g

Fiber: 3g

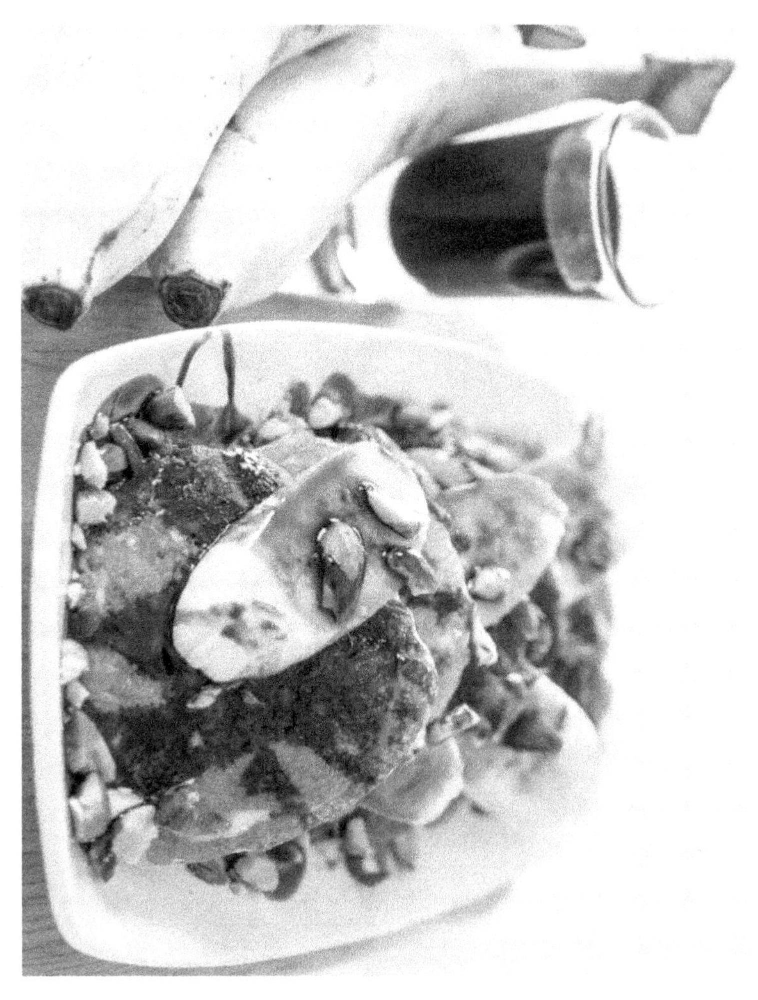

CHAPTER 6: INCORPORATING SUPERFOODS

Quinoa and Kale Salad

Ingredients:

- 1 cup of cooked quinoa
- Kale, chopped
- Cherry tomatoes, sliced
- ½ Avocado
- Walnuts, diced
- Feta cheese (optional)
- Olive oil
- Lemon juice
- Salt and pepper to taste

Preparation:

- In a bowl, combine quinoa, chopped kale, cherry tomatoes, avocado, and walnuts.
- Sprinkle with feta cheese, if desired.
- Drizzle with olive oil and lemon juice.

- Season with salt and pepper to taste.

Nutritional Value (Approx. per serving):

Calories: 350-400

Protein: 10g

Carbohydrates: 30g

Fat: 20g

Fiber: 8g

Sweet Potato and Turmeric Soup:

Ingredients:

- 2 sweet potatoes, peeled and diced
- 1 onion, diced
- 2 carrots, diced
- 1 can of coconut milk
- 1 teaspoon of turmeric powder
- 1 teaspoon of ginger, grated
- Vegetable broth
- Salt and pepper to taste

Preparation:

- Sauté the onion, sweet potatoes, and carrots in a saucepan until tender.
- Stir in the turmeric powder and grated ginger.
- Pour in enough vegetable broth to cover the veggies with coconut milk.
- Cook until the vegetables are soft.
- Blend until smooth, then season with salt and pepper to taste.

Nutritional Value (Approx. per serving):

Calories: 250-300

Protein: 5g

Carbohydrates: 30g

Fat: 15g

Fiber: 6g

Salmon and Quinoa Bowl:

Ingredients:

- Grilled salmon fillet

- 1 cup of cooked quinoa
- Broccoli florets, steamed
- Cherry tomatoes, sliced
- Avocado, sliced
- Pumpkin seeds
- Lemon-tahini dressing

Lemon-tahini dressing:

- 2 tablespoons of tahini
- 1 lemon, juiced
- 1 tablespoon of olive oil
- Salt and pepper to taste

Preparation:

- Combine grilled salmon, cooked quinoa, steamed broccoli, cherry tomatoes, avocado, and pumpkin seeds in a bowl.
- In a small mixing bowl, combine the tahini, lemon juice, olive oil, salt, and pepper.
- Drizzle the dressing over the top of the bowl.

Nutritional Value (Approx. per serving):

Calories: 400-450

Protein: 30g

Carbohydrates: 30g

Fat: 20g

Fiber: 8g

Superfoods for PCOS Management

Polycystic Ovary Syndrome (PCOS) is a hormonal condition that can be controlled with dietary and lifestyle changes. Incorporating nutrient-dense superfoods into your diet can benefit your general health and may aid in the management of PCOS symptoms. Here are some superfoods to consider incorporating into your diet:

Berry:

Antioxidants, vitamins, and fibre are abundant in blueberries, strawberries, raspberries, and blackberries. They can aid in blood sugar management and supply important nutrients.

Leafy Greens:

Folate, iron, and calcium are all found in spinach, kale, and other leafy greens. They are low in calories and high in fibre, making them ideal for weight loss.

Fatty Fish:

Omega-3 fatty acids, which have anti-inflammatory qualities and may help control insulin levels, are abundant in salmon, mackerel, and sardines.

Quinoa:

Quinoa is a protein- and fiber-rich whole grain. It has a low glycemic index, making it an excellent choice for blood sugar management.

Chia Seeds:

Chia seeds include a high concentration of omega-3 fatty acids, fibre, and protein. They can assist to maintain blood sugar levels and provide a sense of fullness.

Turmeric (curcumin):

Turmeric's main ingredient, curcumin, has anti-inflammatory effects. It may aid in the management of inflammation associated with PCOS.

Avocado:

Avocado contains monounsaturated fats, which can help regulate hormones. It also contains important vitamins and minerals.

Cinnamon:

Cinnamon may aid with insulin sensitivity and blood sugar control. Sprinkle it over muesli, yoghurt or smoothies.

Greek yoghurt:

Greek yoghurt has a lot of protein and probiotics. It might be an excellent choice for supporting digestive health and supplying critical minerals.

Nuts and seeds: Nutrients such as omega-3 fatty acids, fibre, and antioxidants are abundant in almonds, walnuts, flaxseeds, and pumpkin seeds.

Broccoli: Is a cruciferous vegetable that is high in fibre and antioxidants. It can help you lose weight and improve your overall health.

Sweet potatoes: Are an excellent source of complex carbs, fibre, and vitamins. When compared to normal potatoes, they have a lower glycemic index.

Lentils: Lentils are high in plant protein, fibre, and vital minerals. They can help to keep blood sugar levels constant.

Green tea: is high in antioxidants and may have anti-inflammatory properties. It can be a healthy substitute for sugary beverages.

It's vital to remember that everyone reacts differently to different meals. Consult a healthcare practitioner or a certified dietitian to develop a personalised dietary plan that meets your unique needs and efficiently manages PCOS symptoms. Maintaining a healthy diet, remaining physically active, and controlling stress are other important components of PCOS treatment.

CHAPTER 7: LIFESTYLE TIPS FOR PCOS

Polycystic Ovary Syndrome (PCOS) is a hormonal disorder that causes irregular periods, cysts on the ovaries, and difficulty becoming pregnant. Lifestyle changes can be quite beneficial in treating PCOS symptoms. Here are some lifestyle suggestions that may be useful:

Eat a Well-Balanced Diet:

Choose entire foods that are high in nutrients. Fruits and vegetables, lean meats, entire grains, and healthy fats should be prioritised.

Portion control is important for weight management since women with PCOS are prone to insulin resistance.

Select Low-Glycemic Foods:

Include meals with a low glycemic index to help manage blood sugar levels. Whole grains, legumes, and non-starchy vegetables are among examples.

Maintain Hydration:

Stay hydrated by drinking plenty of water. Water is crucial for general health and might aid with weight management.

Physical Activity on a Regular Basis:

Exercise on a regular basis to enhance insulin sensitivity and aid with weight management. Aim for at least 150 minutes per week of moderate-intensity aerobic exercise.

Incorporate Strength Training:

In order to gain muscular mass, use strength training workouts. This can assist to boost metabolism and aid in weight loss.

Stress Management:

Yoga, meditation, deep breathing, and mindfulness are all stress-reduction strategies. Chronic stress can aggravate the symptoms of PCOS.

Get Enough Sleep:

Make sure you get adequate rest each night. Aim for 7-9 hours of sleep every night, as inadequate sleep might interfere with hormone control.

Reduce your intake of processed foods and sugars:

Limit your consumption of processed meals, sugary snacks, and beverages. This can lead to insulin resistance and weight gain.

Keep an eye on your carbohydrate intake:

Keep an eye on your carbohydrate consumption and think about integrating complex carbs that give long-lasting energy.

Consider Low-Dairy Alternatives: - Dairy consumption may assist some women with PCOS since it may affect hormonal balance.

Regular Check-ups: Make an appointment with your healthcare practitioner for regular check-ups. It is critical to monitor hormone levels, manage prescriptions, and handle any new concerns.

Birth Control tablets: Some PCOS patients may be prescribed birth control tablets to help regulate their menstrual cycles and manage their symptoms. Consult your healthcare physician to determine the best alternatives for you.

Fertility Planning: If you're thinking about having a baby, consult with your healthcare team to treat PCOS symptoms and optimise fertility.

Seek Help: Connect with support groups or a PCOS-specific healthcare practitioner. Emotional support can help with disease management.

Individualised Approach: - PCOS manifests differently in each individual. Work with healthcare providers to create an individualised strategy that takes into account your specific symptoms, concerns, and goals.

CHAPTER 8: 7-DAY MEAL PLANS

Day 1:

Breakfast:

Greek yogurt parfait with mixed berries, chia seeds, and a drizzle of honey.

Lunch:

Quinoa and vegetable stir-fry with tofu or lean protein.

Snack:

Handful of almonds or walnuts.

Dinner:

Baked salmon with a side of roasted sweet potatoes and steamed broccoli.

Day 2:

Breakfast:

Spinach and feta omelet with whole-grain toast.

Lunch:

Lentil and vegetable soup with a side of mixed greens salad.

Snack:

Apple slices with almond butter.

Dinner:

Grilled chicken breast with quinoa and sautéed kale.

Day 3:

Breakfast:

Smoothie with spinach, mixed berries, Greek yogurt, and a tablespoon of chia seeds.

Lunch:

Whole-grain wrap with hummus, cucumber, tomatoes, and lean turkey or chicken.

Snack:

Vegetable sticks with Hummus

Dinner:

Stir-fried shrimp with broccoli and cauliflower rice.

Day 4:

Breakfast:

Overnight oats with almond milk, topped with sliced banana and a sprinkle of cinnamon.

Lunch:

Quinoa salad with chickpeas, cherry tomatoes, cucumber, and a lemon-tahini dressing.

Snack:

Cottage cheese with pineapple chunks.

Dinner:

Turkey and vegetable kebabs with a side of quinoa.

Day 5:

Breakfast:

Avocado and tomato toast on whole-grain bread.

Lunch:

Spinach and strawberry salad with grilled chicken and a balsamic vinaigrette.

Snack:

Handful of mixed nuts.

Dinner:

Baked cod with asparagus and a side of wild rice.

Day 6:

Breakfast:

Whole-grain pancakes with fresh berries and a dollop of Greek yogurt.

Lunch:

Vegetable and lentil curry with brown rice.

Snack:

Green tea and a handful of dark chocolate-covered almonds.

Dinner:

Quinoa-stuffed bell peppers with lean ground turkey and black beans.

Breakfast:

Scrambled eggs with sautéed spinach, cherry tomatoes, and whole-grain toast.

Lunch:

Greek salad with grilled shrimp.

Snack:

Sliced pear with a sprinkle of cinnamon.

Dinner:

Baked chicken laps with sweet potato wedges and green beans.

CHAPTER 9: CONCLUSION

It is critical to recognise the transforming effect of adopting a comprehensive approach to controlling Polycystic Ovary Syndrome (PCOS). Navigating the dietary landscape with an emphasis on nutrient-dense, balanced meals addresses not just the unique nutritional demands associated with PCOS, but also promotes a good connection with food.

This cookbook aims to empower persons who have just been diagnosed with PCOS by offering a wide range of recipes designed to assist hormonal balance, weight control, and general well-being. The cookbook aims to transform regular meals into a source of health and healing by adding an extensive variety of whole foods, superfoods, and PCOS-friendly ingredients.

Furthermore, the path described in these pages continues beyond the kitchen, urging people to adopt lifestyle changes such as physical exercise, stress management, and mindful eating. Recognising that everyone's experience with PCOS is different, the cookbook promotes flexibility and personalisation in meal planning, allowing people to adjust recipes to their tastes and nutritional preferences.

In summary, "The Complete PCOS Cookbook for the Newly Diagnosed" is a thorough handbook that not only provides tasty meals but also fosters a sense of empowerment and control. It is a tool that enables people to take control of their health, make educated decisions, and live a full and active life despite the obstacles of PCOS. Finally, this cookbook is a monument to the strength of persons dealing with PCOS, giving them with the tools they need to begin on a path towards better health and well-being.

BE HEALTHY!

MEAL PLANNER

DAILY

DATE

BREAKFAST

LUNCH

SNACK

DINNER

NOTES

ITEMS LIST

MEAL PLANNER

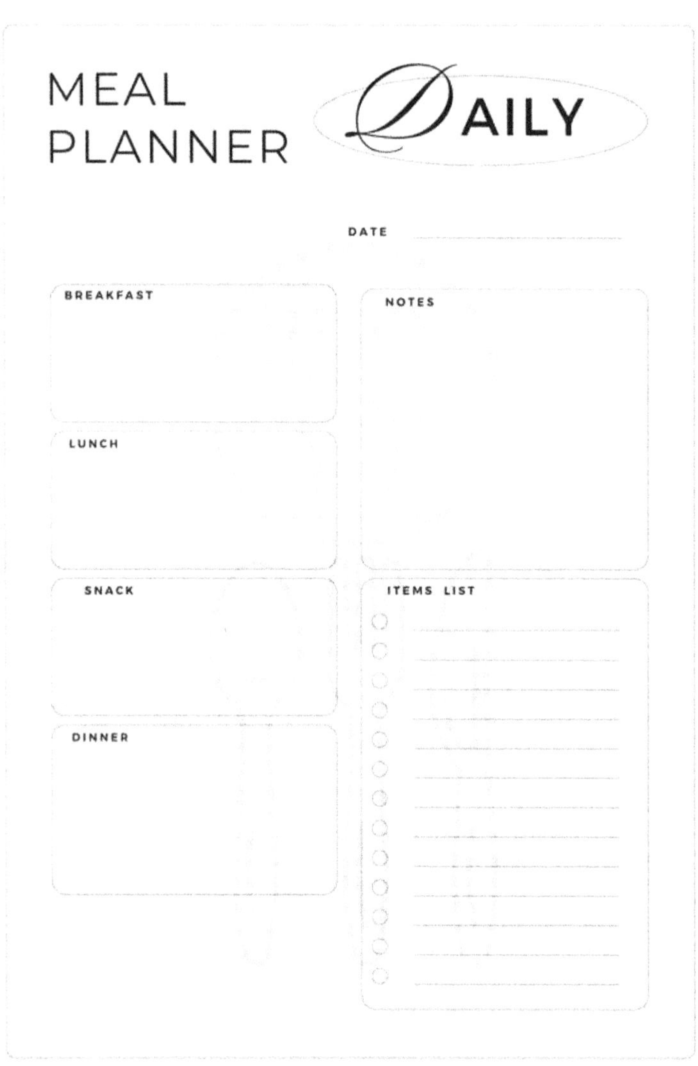

MEAL PLANNER

DAILY

DATE

BREAKFAST

NOTES

LUNCH

SNACK

ITEMS LIST

DINNER

MEAL
PLANNER

Daily

DATE

BREAKFAST

LUNCH

SNACK

DINNER

NOTES

ITEMS LIST

MEAL PLANNER

*D*AILY

DATE

BREAKFAST

NOTES

LUNCH

SNACK

ITEMS LIST

DINNER

MEAL PLANNER

DAILY

DATE

BREAKFAST

LUNCH

SNACK

DINNER

NOTES

ITEMS LIST

MEAL PLANNER

DAILY

DATE

BREAKFAST

NOTES

LUNCH

SNACK

ITEMS LIST

DINNER